Lynda Aoudia

BI-RADS mammography glossary

Lynda Aoudia

BI-RADS mammography glossary

Step by step

ScienciaScripts

Imprint
Any brand names and product names mentioned in this book are subject to trademark, brand or patent protection and are trademarks or registered trademarks of their respective holders. The use of brand names, product names, common names, trade names, product descriptions etc. even without a particular marking in this work is in no way to be construed to mean that such names may be regarded as unrestricted in respect of trademark and brand protection legislation and could thus be used by anyone.

Cover image: www.ingimage.com

This book is a translation from the original published under ISBN 978-620-6-71380-7.

Publisher:
Sciencia Scripts
is a trademark of
Dodo Books Indian Ocean Ltd. and OmniScriptum S.R.L publishing group

120 High Road, East Finchley, London, N2 9ED, United Kingdom
Str. Armeneasca 28/1, office 1, Chisinau MD-2012, Republic of Moldova, Europe
Printed at: see last page
ISBN: 978-620-7-67302-5

Mammography BI-RADS glossary: step by step

Lynda AOUDIA

Foreword

Since 1993, the American College of Radiology (ACR) has published the BI-RADS "Breast Imaging-Reporting and Data System", which provides an accurate description of mammographic abnormalities, with a detailed lexicon of terms, and a precise mammographic report with evaluation categories, making it easier for corresponding physicians to understand the reports and compare them with previous examinations. A latest American version of BI-RADS entitled "BI-RADS® Atlas" was published by the ACR in 2013,

Prof. Lynda AOUDIA

Table of contents

Introduction

The BI-RADS *(Breast Imaging Reporting and Data System)* developed by the *American College of Radiology* (ACR) in collaboration with other organizations, such as the *Food and Drug* Administration (FDA) and the *National Cancer Institute.* The initial aim of this tool was to improve the quality of breast cancer screening campaigns, while standardizing mammography reporting through the use of a common lexicon, resulting in more appropriate action and easier follow-up. This classification has a number of advantages: it guides the radiologist in the description of mammographic abnormalities, trying to reduce inter-observer discordance and homogenize descriptive terms, resulting in a classification that is as reproducible as possible and appropriate action to be taken.

Classically, this assessment is based on various anomalies (mass, calcifications, architectural disorganizations, "special" cases, associated findings), according to which these anomalies will be classified into one of six categories depending on the degree of suspicion of malignancy, which will subsequently enable us to propose appropriate management [1] (Table 1).

Table 1. BI-RADS mammography evaluation categories

BI-RADS 0	Incomplete assessment requiring further imaging
BI-RADS 1	Normal mammography
BI-RADS 2	Benign anomaly.
BI-RADS 3	Anomaly probably benign, with a risk of malignancy < 2%, short-term monitoring is recommended.
BI-RADS 4	Suspicious abnormality, with a probability of malignancy of between 3% and 95%, requiring histological analysis. • 4a = low probability, • 4b = moderate probability, • 4c = high probability.
BI-RADS 5	Highly suspicious anomaly, with probability of malignancy > 95%, requiring surgical removal.
BI-RADS 6	Known histological result: proven malignancy.

Anatomical reminder

1. Breast anatomy

The breast is a globular organ occupying the anterosuperior part of the thorax. It is located above the pectoralis muscle, which provides support [2]. It consists mainly of a mammary gland, supportive connective tissue and adipose tissue, all covered by the skin. The apex of the breast is represented by the nipple surrounded by the areola (fig. 1). It is made up of some fifteen main galactophores, each delimiting a lobe. The milk ducts open into the nipple at the level of the milk pores, after dilating slightly to form a lactiferous sinus.

Thin fibrous partitions separate the lobes, extending from the anterior surface of the gland into the dermis to form Cooper's ligaments and Duret's ridges (fig. 1).

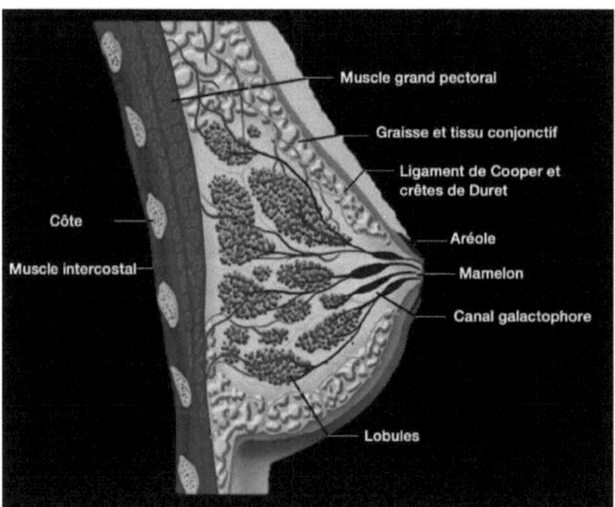

Fig. 1. anatomical structure of the breast.

2. Galactophoric tree

The breast is made up of some fifteen main milk ducts, which end in a nipple pore. These main ducts, after a dilatation known as the lactiferous sinus, branch out into secondary ducts of medium and small caliber up to the Ductulo-Lobular Terminal Unit (DLTU).

This UDTL consists of an extra- and intra-lobular terminal galactophore and a lobule made up of ten or so alveoli called acini. The UDTL is embedded in a loose connective tissue known as pallaeal tissue. All this tissue is surrounded by adipose tissue (fig. 2). The alveolus or acinus takes the form of a small, rounded, microscopic sac. It is made up of two types of cells: secretory epithelial cells and myoepithelial cells responsible for contraction, resting on a basement membrane in direct contact with the blood vessels.

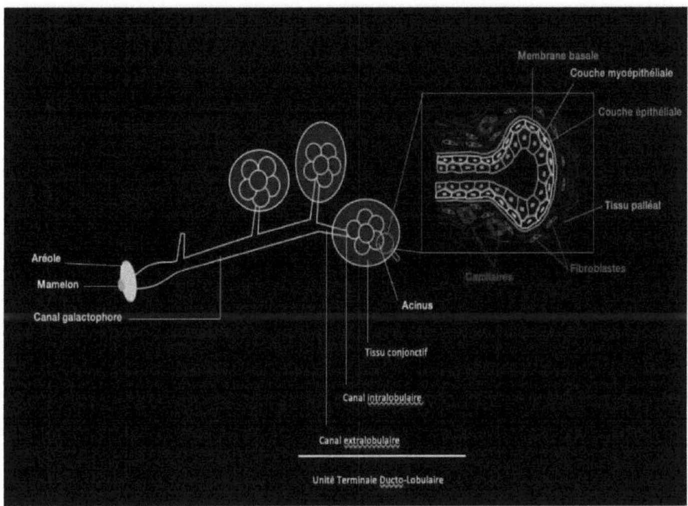

Fig. 2: Schematic representation of the ducto-lobular end unit.

Mammography technique

Mammography is the reference radiological examination for screening for breast cancer, the leading cause of death in women.

Mammographic images must be optimized in terms of spatial resolution, contrast and noise. A number of technical criteria need to be taken into account, including high contrast for good visualization of microcalcifications. The radiation spectrum must be broad, to adapt to varying breast densities, and the radiation dose must be minimal, especially in young patients.

1. Impact

Positioning the breast is a fundamental step in mammography, and the technique must be beyond reproach. The aim is to radiograph the entire mammary gland, including the deep planes. Positioning is the key to obtaining optimal images, essential for interpretation, and meeting a number of quality criteria [3].

1.1. Fundamental impacts

1.1.1. Cranio-caudal or frontal incidence

The X-ray beam approaches the breast craniocaudally (fig. 3).

The difficulty of the front view lies in the absence of visualization of the deep mammary planes, and it is important to engage as much posterior mammary tissue as possible.

The criteria for successful incidence are (fig. 4):

- The breast is at the center of the image.

- The gland is well spread out.

- The nipple is at its zenith [4].

- No folds or overlaps.

The pectoralis muscle is visible in almost 30% of cases, and its presence on the x-ray allows optimum depth gain [3].

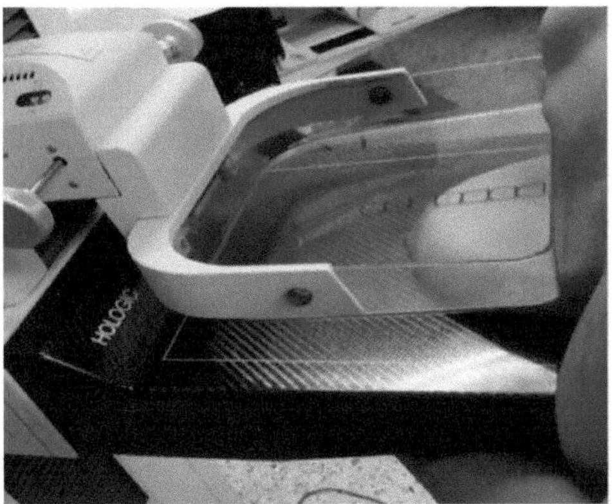

Fig. 3. Front view.

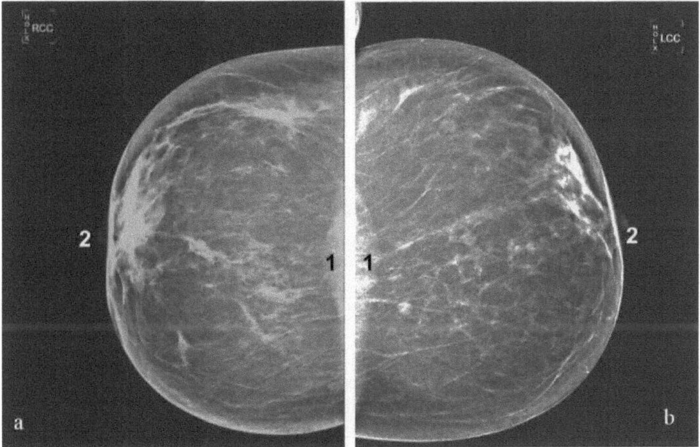

Fig. 4: Quality criteria for frontal incidence. Mammographic images. (a) Right face. (b) Left face. Pectoral muscle (1), nipple at zenith (2).

1.1.2. 45° external oblique incidence°

This allows the breast to be studied in its long axis, and a maximum

amount of breast tissue to be analyzed [5]. The stand is tilted at a strict 45°°
to ensure reproducible incidence (fig. 5).

The difficulty with this incidence is to evenly compress the pectoral
muscle, the breast and the submammary fold.

The criteria for successful incidence are (fig. 6)

-   The pectoral muscle is visible up to halfway up the image [6].

-   The nipple is at its zenith, opposite the tip of the pectoral muscle [5].

-   Presence of abdominal wall skin fold [4].

-   The long axis of the breast tends towards the horizontal.

-   Presence of the "open" submammary fold, perfectly clear of the
    abdominal wall [7].

-   No folds or overlaps.

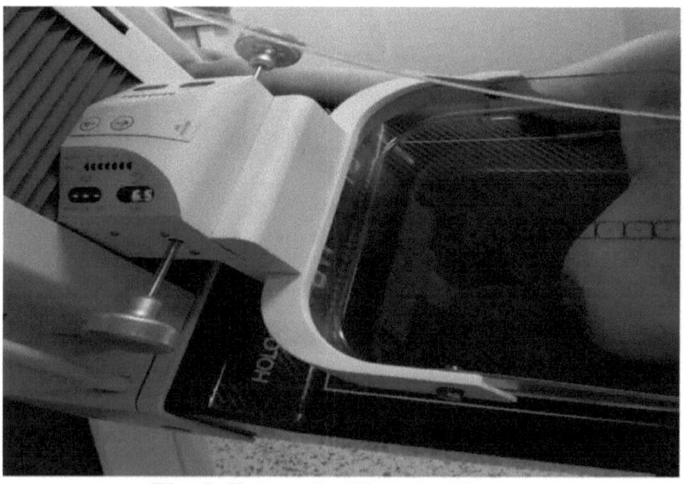

Fig. 5. External oblique incidence.

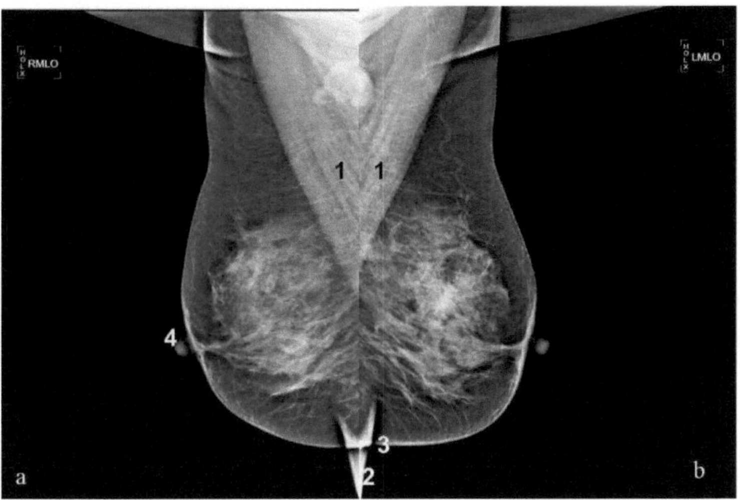

Fig. 6: Quality criteria for external oblique incidence. Mammographic images (a) Right oblique (b) Left oblique. Pectoral muscle (1), abdominal wall skin fold (2), open sub-mammary fold (3), nipple at zenith (4).

1.2. Additional impacts

They are always carried out in addition to the fundamental impacts.

1.2.1. Profile incidence

It is useful for determining the precise location of a lesion. It can also be used to highlight the sloping nature of microcalcifications.

1.2.2. Localized centric view

It can be used to analyze the contours of a nodule or stellate image, or to eliminate a constructed image (fig. 7).

1.2.3. Enlarged centered shot

It enables microcalcifications visible on standard images to be enlarged for detailed analysis (number, appearance, organization, etc.) (fig. 8).

1.2.4. Other impacts

Axillary extension, Cleopatra incidence, staggered frontal incidence, tangential cliché, Eklund maneuver [8-11].

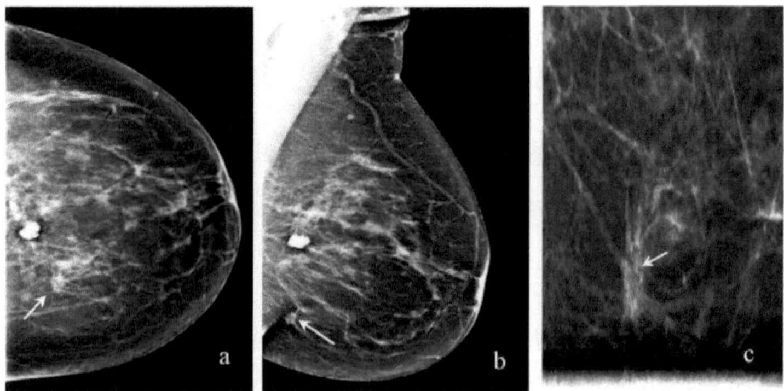

Fig. 7. localized centric view. (a) Front view. Mass with indistinct contours (arrow). (b) External oblique view. Mass in the sub mammary fold with poorly defined contours (arrow). (c). View centred on the mass. Mass with spiculated contours, BIRADS 5 (arrow).

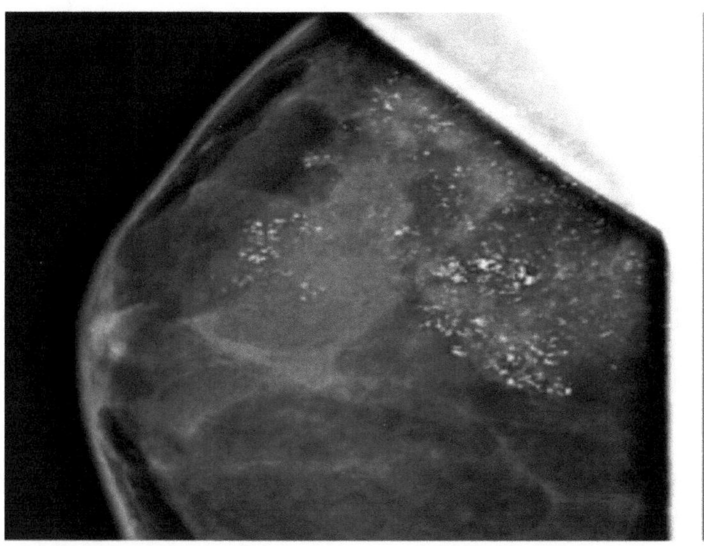

Fig. 8. Enlarged centric view. Magnification of a focus of microcalcifications.

Anatomy - mammography correlations [12-14]

Mammography produces a two-dimensional projection of the breast. The mammographic image is a superimposition of all the tissues making up the breast, varying according to the proportion of the different constituents (parenchymal tissue, adipose tissue, connective tissue), age and hormonal impregnation.

The different elements visualized by mammography, from surface to depth.

1.3. The skin covering

The cutaneous plane is a dense border, approximately 1 mm thick (fig. 9); it is thicker at the areola and in the sub-mammary region. Skin pores may be visible as punctiform blisters.

1.4. The nipple

The nipple is dense on mammography, cylindrical-conical in shape, about 1cm long, and should be located outside the gland contours (fig. 9). The nipple may become invaginated or hypertrophied.

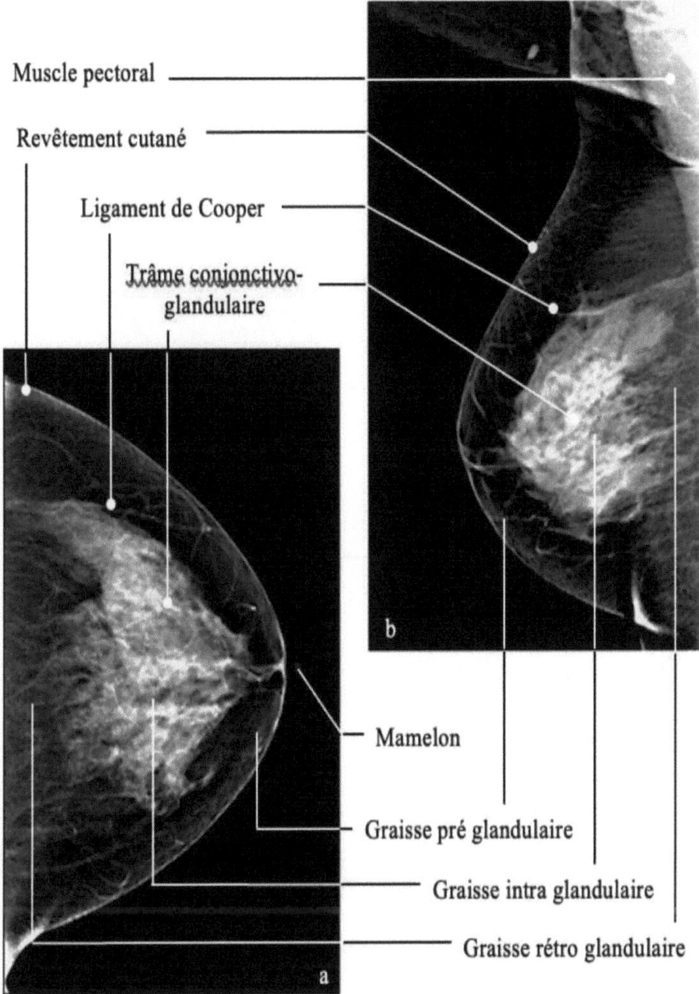

Fig. 9. Breast constitution. Mammography, (a) craniocaudal incidence, (b) oblique incidence.

1.5. Glandular tissue

Imaging of the breast contents depends on the glandular component. Lobular elements are visible thanks to the contrast of the intralobular connective tissue and, on mammography, appear as small, fuzzy micronodular opacities [15]. Galactophore ducts are not spontaneously visible on mammography, except in the case of very fatty environments and ductal dilatation (fig. 10).

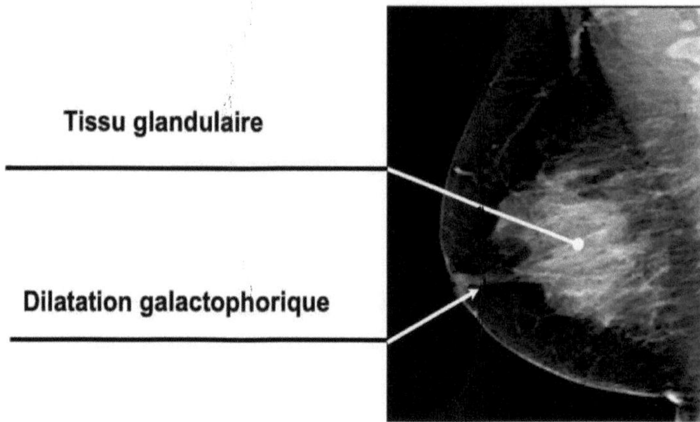

Fig. 10. Galactophoric dilatation. Mammography, incidence

1.6. Connective tissue

The connective tissue, radiopaque, is sparse and its opacity is confused with that of the glandular tissue. Cooper's ligaments appear as linear or arciform opacities. They are generally visible on oblique or profile mammography. Cooper's ligaments are prominent in subcutaneous adipose tissue, along the upper edge of the parenchyma (fig. 9).

1.7. Adipose tissue

Adipose tissue, radiolucent on mammography. A subcutaneous, preglandular fatty space is crossed by Cooper's ligaments, and a retroglandular fatty space separates the gland from the pectoral muscle. This is the *no-man's-land* zone described by Tabar [15,16] (fig. 9).

1.8. The muscles

On the craniocaudal view, the pectoral muscle is inconsistently projected forward of the chest wall in the form of a half-moon. On the medio-lateral oblique view, the pectoralis muscle is seen as a concave structure behind the retroglandular fat (fig. 9).

The sternal muscle is located in internal projection on craniocaudal incidence, rarely visible in 1% of patients (fig. 11).

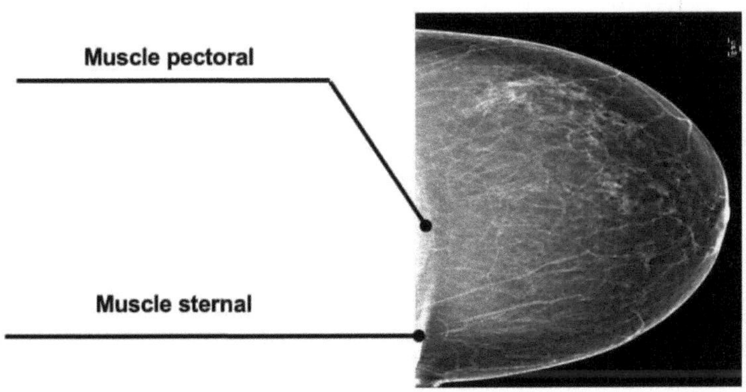

Fig. 11. visualization of the sternal muscle projection. Mammography, frontal view.

1.9. Vessels

Vessels can be visualized, especially if the contrast is fatty. They appear as dense, ribbon-like structures. Veins are larger than arteries. Occasionally, vessels can be identified by atheromatous parietal calcifications (fig. 12).

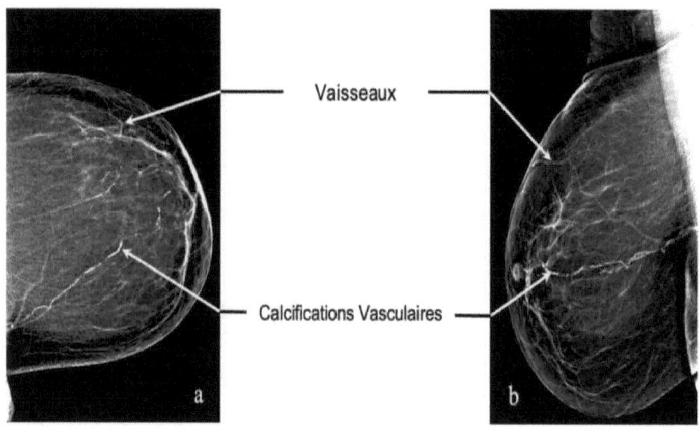

Fig. 12. Vascularization. (a) Mammography, craniocaudal incidence, (b) oblique incidence.

1.7. Lymphatic vessels

Lymphatic vessels are absent in normal breasts. Nodes are detected intra-mammary in 5% of normal mammograms [17] (fig. 13). They have the appearance of a kidney-shaped or dense coffee-bean structure with a clear fat center, and are usually located along the vessels (fig. 13).

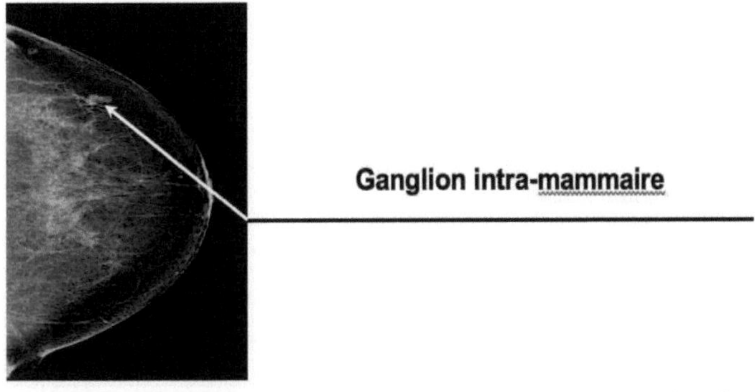

Fig. 13. Intramammary ganglion, with clear center, projecting from a vascular structure. Mammogram, frontal view.

BI-RADS Glossary

1. Assessment of breast density

The different mammographic aspects result from the variable proportion between fibrous and fatty elements in the breast. The earliest classification was described by Wolfe in 1967 [18], determining four types of glandular density (N1, P1, P2, NY), with type N1 corresponding to a totally fatty glandular structure through to type NY, which corresponds to a totally dense glandular structure. The American College of Radiology has adapted these different categories in Breast Imaging Reporting into 4 types from "a" to "d" [1] (fig. 14):

- Type "a": Breasts almost entirely fatty; glandular tissue less than 25%.
- Type "b": Breasts composed of scattered areas of fibro-glandular density, with glandular tissue at around 25-50%.
- Type "c": heterogeneously dense breasts, which may mask small masses; glandular tissue between 51 and 75% approximately.
- Type "d": Extremely dense breasts, reducing mammography sensitivity; glandular tissue more than 75%.

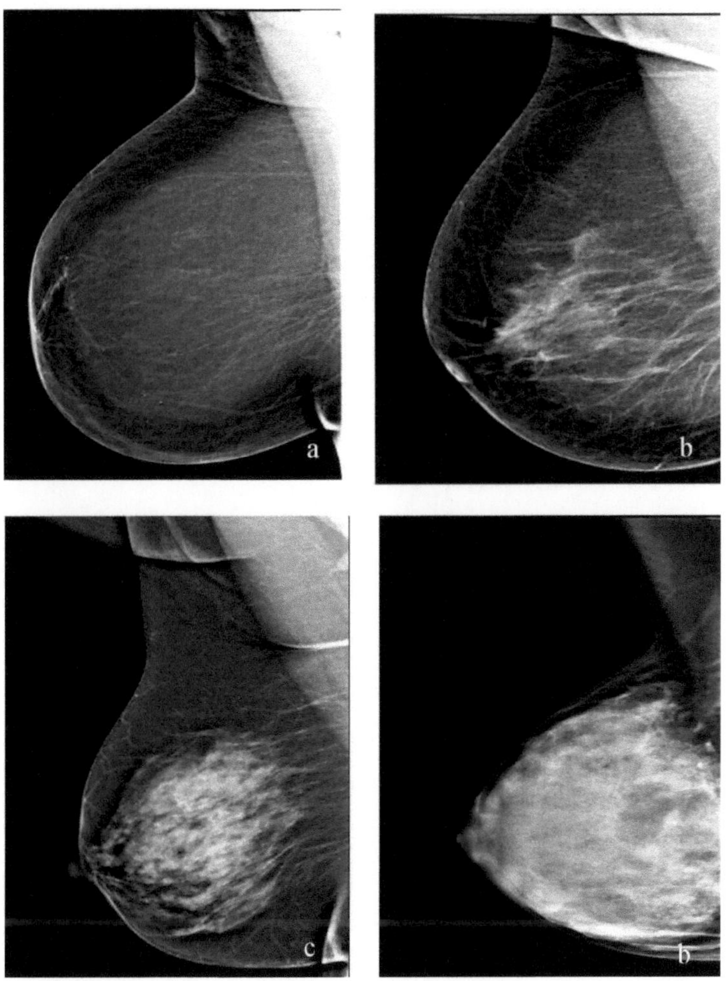

Fig. 14. Breast density. Mammography, oblique incidence. (a): almost entirely fatty, type a; (b): scattered patches of fibroglandular tissue, type b; (c): heterogeneous dense breast, type c; (d): extremely dense breast, type d.

2. Lesion description according to BI-RADS lexicon

2.1. Weights

A mass is a mammographic image occupying a volume in space, seen on two different views. If a mass is seen on a single view, it is considered as a density asymmetry until its three-dimensional nature is confirmed. The mass should be described in terms of its shape, contours and density. The characteristics of masses with their malignancy score, according to BIRADS 2013, are summarized in Table 2

2.1.1. Shape

The shape can be :
- **Oval**: an ellipsoidal or ovoid mass (fig. 15).
- **Round:** a spherical, ball-shaped, circular or globular mass (fig. 16).
- **Irregular:** a mass whose shape is neither round nor oval (fig. 17).

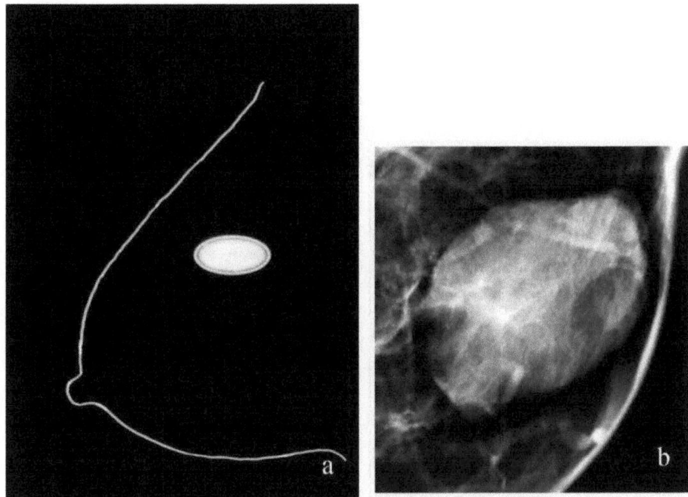

Fig. 15. Oval shape. (a) Diagram. (b) Mammogram.

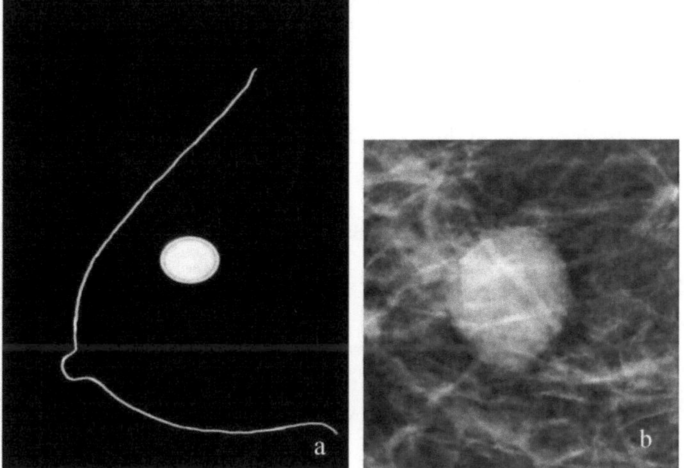

Fig. 16: Round shape (a) Diagram. (b) Mammogram.

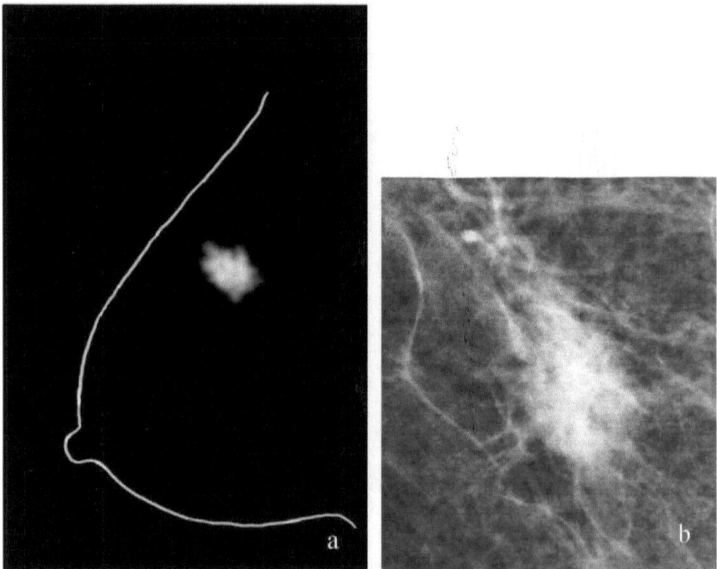

Fig. 17. Irregular shape. (a) Diagram. (b) Mammogram.

2.1.2. Contours

They modify the shape of the mass. They can be :

- **Circumscribed, well-defined or sharp**: contours are clearly delineated, seen over at least 75% of the mass circumference, the rest being masked by adjacent tissue with an abrupt transition between lesion and adjacent tissue (fig. 18).
- **Microlobulated**: characterized by the presence of short serrations creating small undulations (fig. 19).
- **Masked**: the contours are hidden over more than 25% of the circumference of the mass by adjacent or superimposed glandular tissue, without this appearance being considered suspicious (fig. 20).
- **Indistinct or poorly defined**: this raises the suspicion of infiltration. This appearance is unlikely to be due to an overlay of normal breast tissue (fig. 21).

-   **Spiculated**: a mass with extensions, highly suggestive of malignancy (fig. 22).

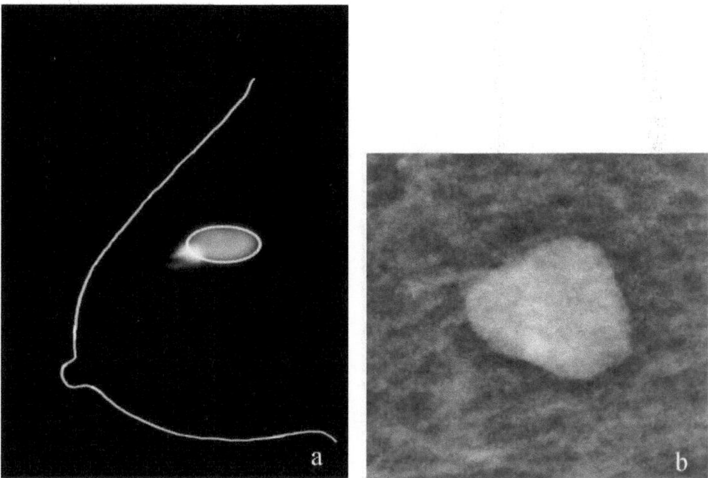

Fig. 18. circumscribed contours (a) diagram. (b) Mammogram. Clear contours, seen over 75%.

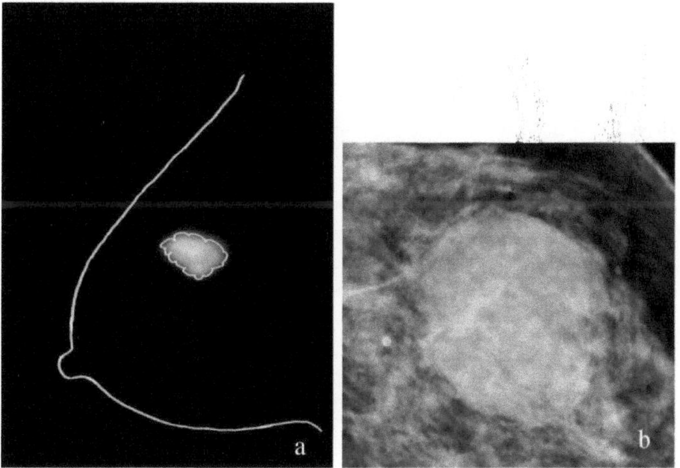

Fig. 19. Microlobulated contours. (a) Diagram. (b) Mammogram. Contours have small undulations.

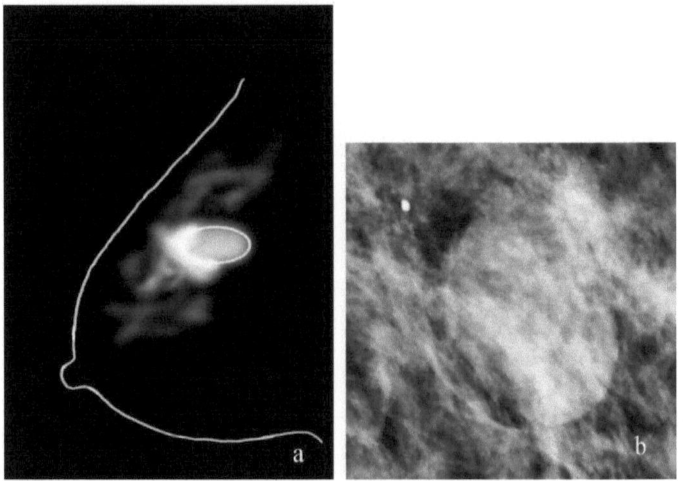

Fig. 20. Masked contours. (a) Diagram. (b) Mammogram. More than 25% of contours hidden.

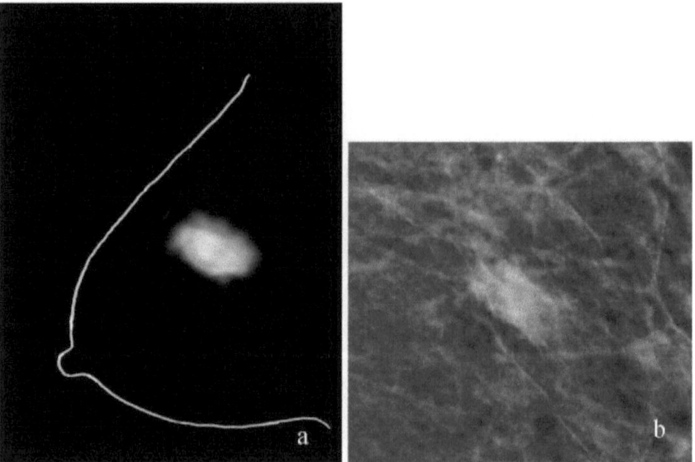

Fig. 21. indistinct contours (a) Diagram. (b) Mammogram. Poorly defined contours.

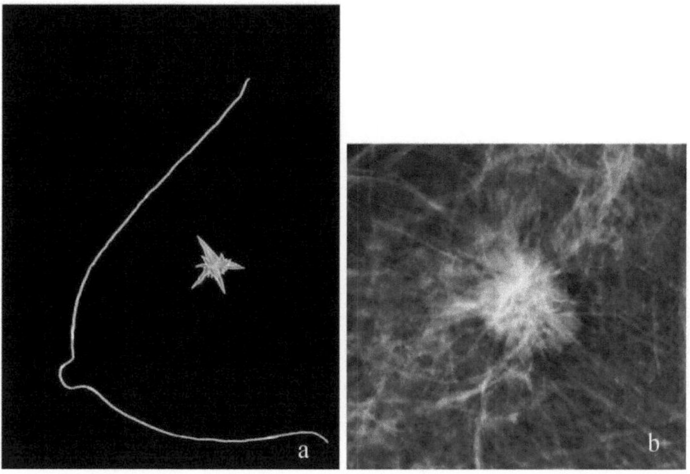

Fig. 22. Spiculated contours. (a) Diagram. (b) Mammogram. Contours show extensions

2.1.2. Density

This term is used to define the attenuation of X-rays by the lesion compared with the attenuation expected from an equivalent volume of fibro-glandular tissue. Most breast cancers appear as a mass with a density equal to or greater than that of breast tissue. It is rare for breast cancer to be of lesser density. The different types of mass density are (fig. 23) :

- Hyperdense: a mass denser than adjacent breast tissue.
- Isodense or intermediate density: a mass of the same density as adjacent breast tissue.
- Hypodense: low-density mass with no fat content
- Radio-transparent or clear: includes all fat-containing masses such as oily cyst, lipoma and galactocele, as well as mixed masses such as hamartoma.

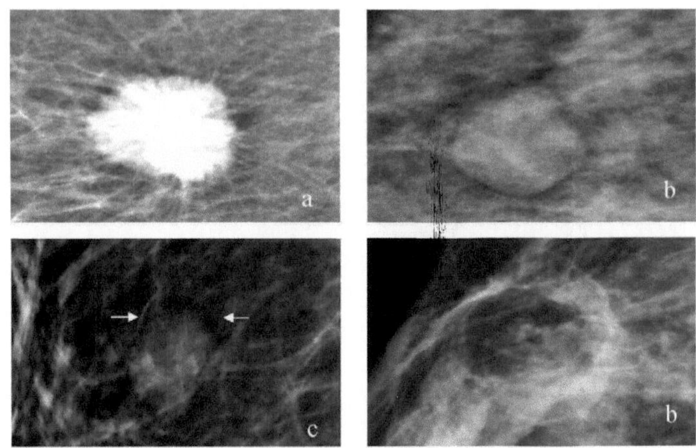

Fig. 23. Mass density: (a) hyperdense, (b) isodense, (c) hypodense (arrows), (d) fatty.

Table 2. Mass characteristics and malignancy scores according to BI-RADS 2013.				
	Probably benign			**Probably clever**
Shape	Oval	Round		Irregular
Contours	Well circumscribed (> 75%)	Masked (> 25%)	Microlobulated	Indistincts	Spiculated
Density	Adipose (PPV= 0%)	Weak or isodense (PPV = 22%)		Strong (PPV= 70%)
BI-RADS (VPP)	BI-RADS 3 (< 2%)	BI-RADS 4a (< 2 and > 10%)	BI-RADS 4b (> 10 and < 50%)	BI-RADS 4c or 5 (> 50%)

2.2. Calcifications

The BI-RADS classification breaks down intramammary calcifications into two types, essentially taking into account their morphology and distribution:
- typically benign calcifications.
- suspicious calcifications. The degree of suspicion of malignancy is increased by the distribution and size of the focus.

2.2.1. Calcification morphology

2.2.1.1. Typically benign calcifications

Benign calcifications, such as cystic "ring" calcifications, vascular calcifications, skin calcifications and so on. They are generally regular, with smooth edges, round if their size is between 0.5 and 1 mm, and punctiform if their size is less than 0.5 mm.

• Skin calcifications

Calcium deposits with clear centers, often pathognomonic, they are usually observed along the submammary fold, in the para-sternal, axillary and areolar regions.

In the case of unusual forms, tangential incidence can be used to confirm their subcutaneous topography (fig. 24).

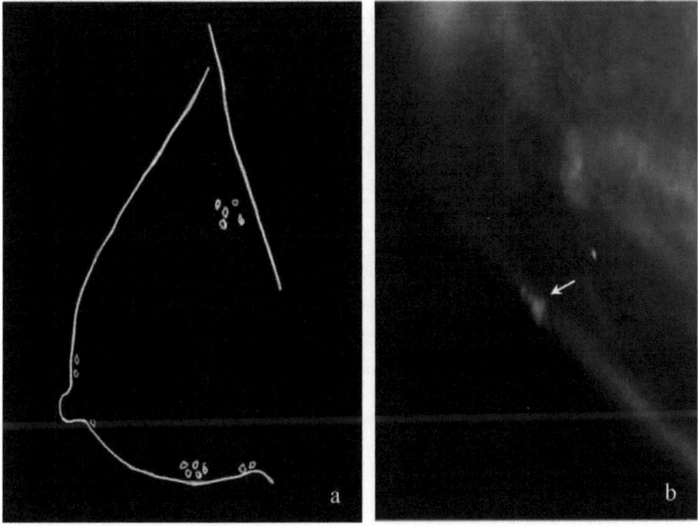

Fig. 24. Cutaneous calcifications. (a) Diagram. (b) Mammogram, tangential view. Cutaneous calcifications (arrow).

- # Vascular calcifications

Rail or linear calcifications, clearly associated with tubular structures (fig. 25).

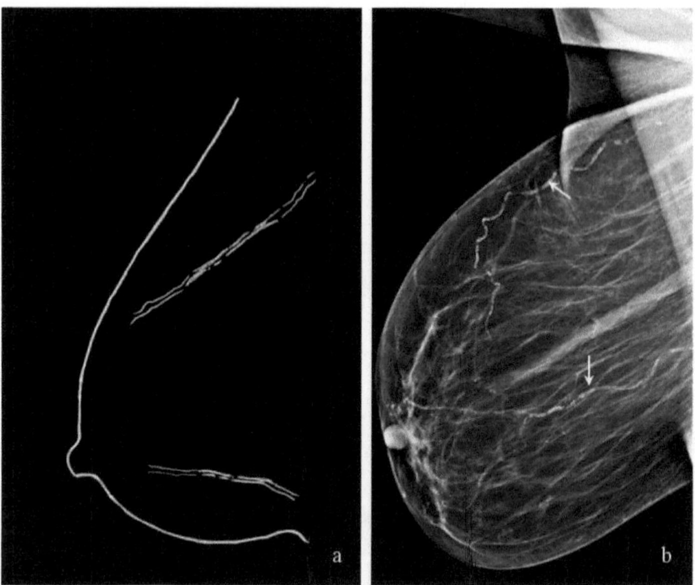

Fig. 25. Vascular calcifications. (a) Schematic diagram. (b) Oblique mammographic view. Rail-like calcifications (arrow).

• Coarse calcifications or Coralliformes

These are large calcifications, over 2-3 mm in diameter, generally secondary to involution of a fibroadenoma (fig. 26, 27).

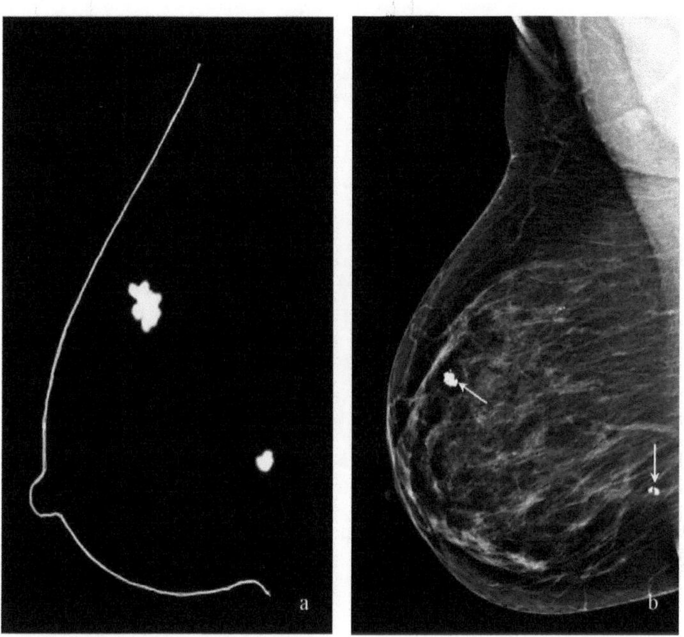

Fig. 26. coralliform calcifications (a) Diagram. (b) Mammogram, oblique view. Large calcifications (arrows).

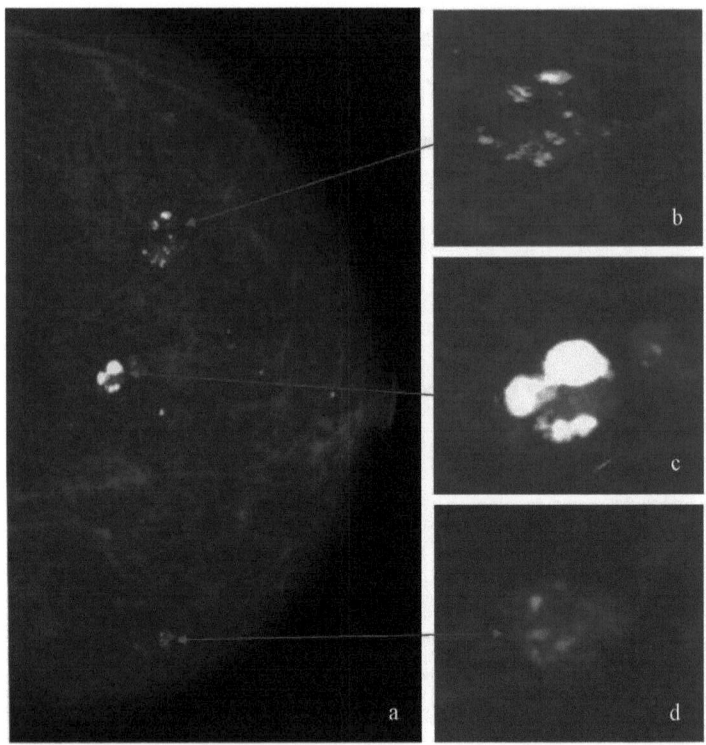

Fig. 27. Coralliform calcifications (a) Mammogram, front view (b+c+d) Enlargements. Calcifications of fibroadenoma in involution.

• **Large rod calcifications**

These are secretory calcifications associated with ductal ectasia, forming smooth-edged, sometimes discontinuous, rods of supramillimetric size. These calcifications may have a clear center if the calcium deposit is in the wall of the galactophore (fig. 28). Their distribution is ductal towards the nipple, and most often bilateral. They are often found in patients over 60 years of age.

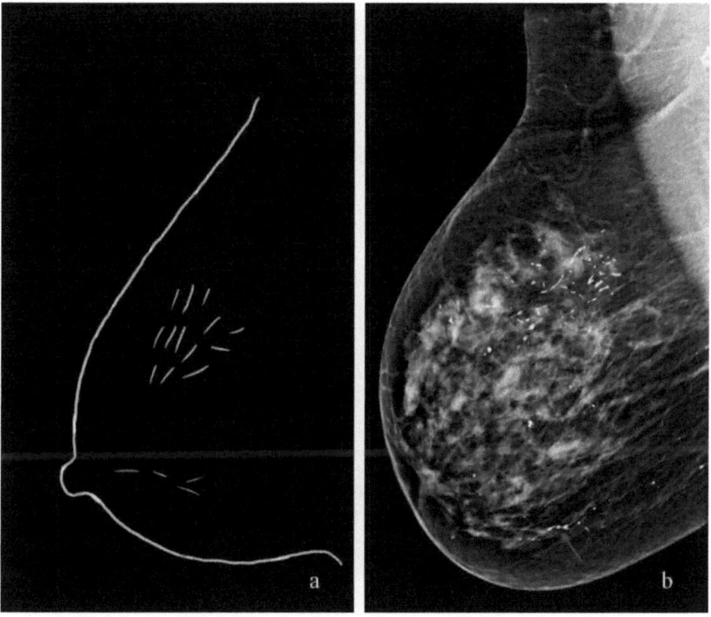

Fig. 28. (a) Schematic diagram. (b) Oblique mammogram. Linear calcifications moving towards the nipple (arrows).

• **Round calcifications**

Round calcifications are often multiple and vary in size. They are considered benign when they are scattered. When they are small, less than 1 mm, they frequently correspond to calcium deposits in the lobular acini (fig. 29). When they are smaller than 0.5 mm, we use the term punctiform. Usually benign, a cluster of microcalcifications is more suspicious and may require surveillance if it has appeared, or if it is present on the same side as a breast cancer (fig. 30).

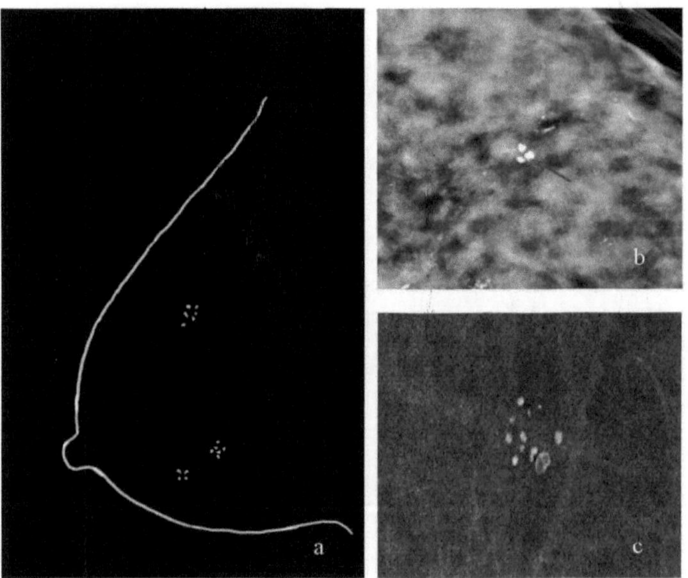

Fig. 29. Round calcifications. (a) Diagram. (b+c) Mammogram. Clusters of round calcifications (arrows).

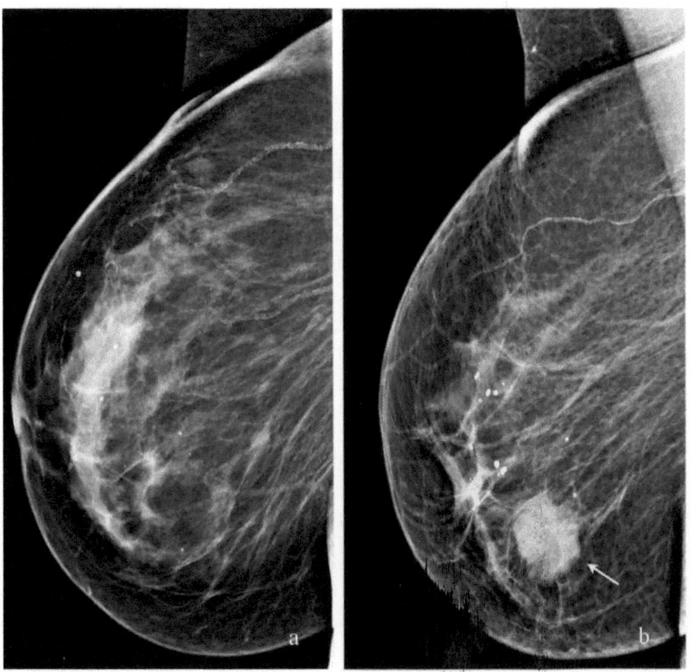

Fig. 30. Round calcifications. (a+b) Mammogram. (a) Scattered round calcifications. (b) Round calcifications associated with an adjacent suspicious mass (arrow).

• Calcifications with clear centers

Calcifications ranging in size from a millimetre to a centimetre, corresponding to cytosteatonecrosis calcifications or calcified ductal debris. They are round or oval with a smooth surface and clear center, with a thicker wall than eggshell calcifications (fig. 31).

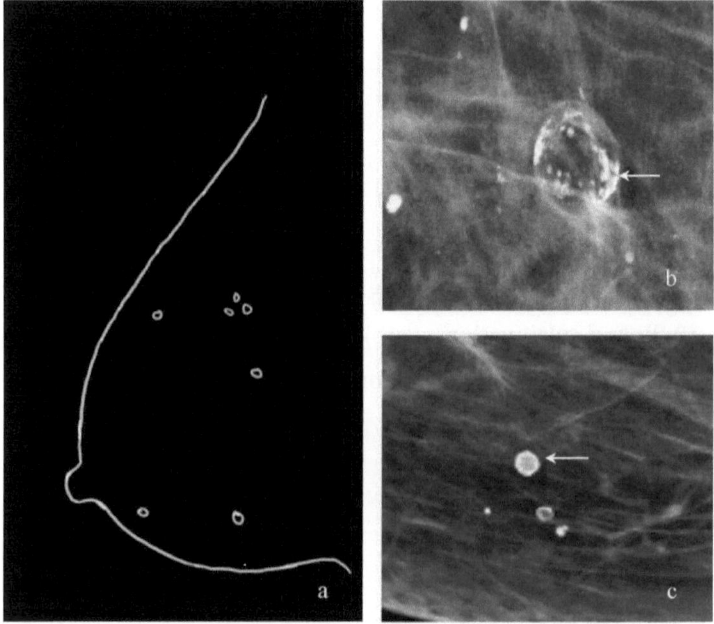

Fig. 31. Calcifications with clear centers (a) Diagram. (b+c) Mammogram.

Round calcifications with smooth surfaces and clear centers (arrows).

• **Eggshell" or parietal calcifications**

These are very fine calcifications with the appearance of a calcium deposit on the surface of a sphere. These deposits are very fine (generally less than 1 mm thick).

The two main etiologies are :

- cyst wall calcifications (fig. 32);

- cytosteatonecrosis (fig. 33).

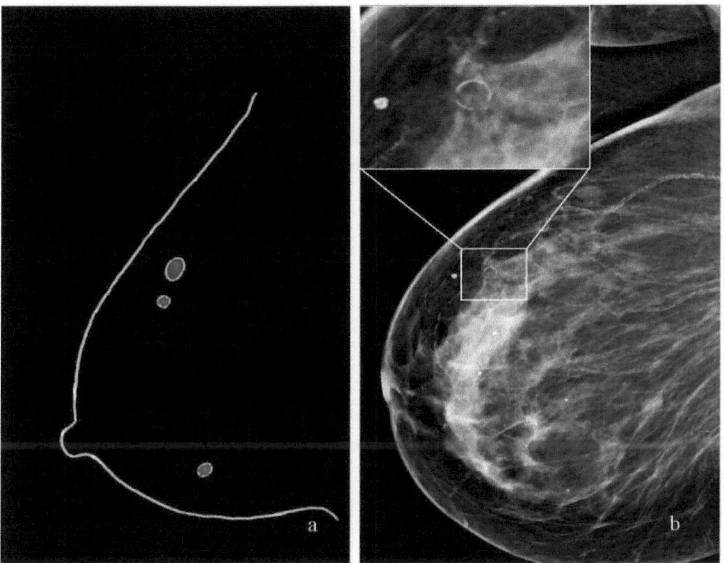

Fig. 32 Eggshell calcifications (a) Diagram. (b) Mammogram.
Calcifications with calcium deposits on the surface of a cystic wall.

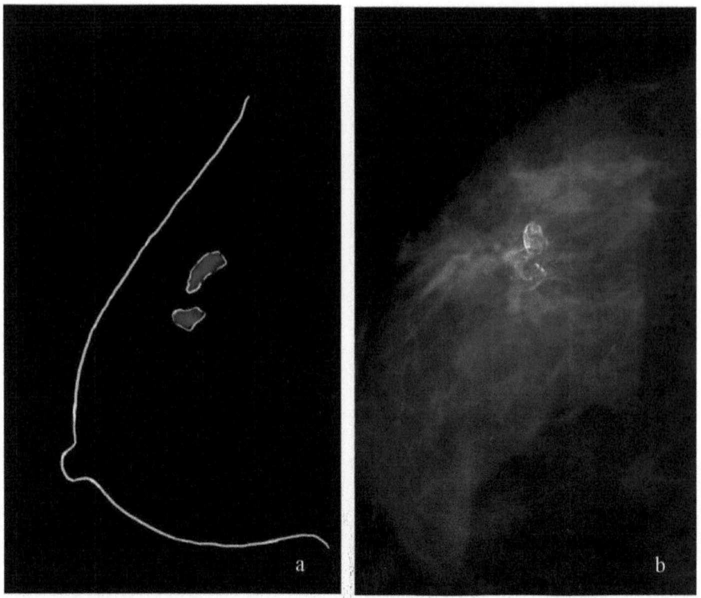

Fig. 33 Eggshell calcifications (a) Diagram. (b) Mammogram. Calcifications with calcium deposits on the surface of a cytosteonecrosis lesion (arrows).

• Calcium milk-type calcifications

They are secondary to intracystic sedimentation of calcified secretion
products. On mammographic views from the front, they appear as
amorphous deposits with blurred boundaries. Strict profile views, on the
other hand, show clear, semilunar, crescent-shaped or curvilinear deposits
with an upper concavity, or linear deposits forming the sloping part of the
cysts (fig. 34).

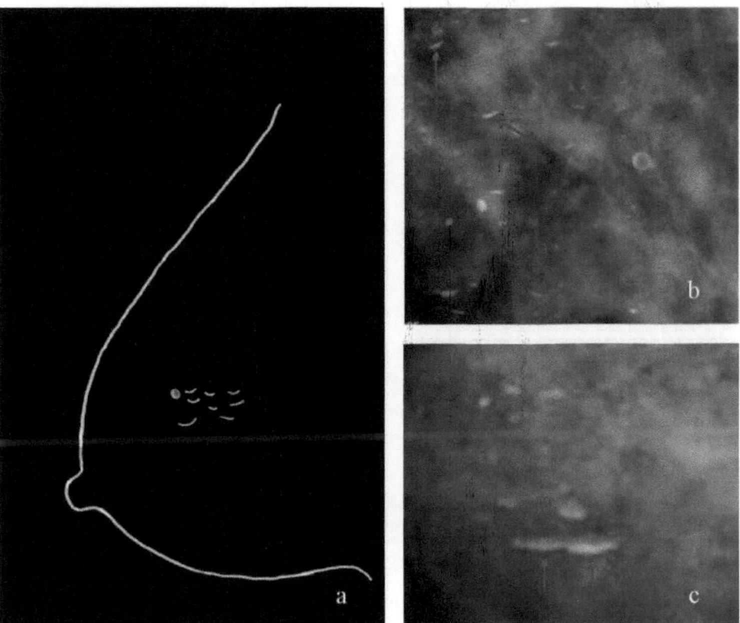

Fig. 34: Calcium milk-type calcifications (a) Diagram. (b+c)
Mammogram. Curvilinear calcifications with upper concavity (arrows).

• Calcified sutures

These calcifications correspond to calcium deposits on suture material. They are more frequent in the irradiated breast. They appear as linear calcifications following the path of the sutures (fig. 35).

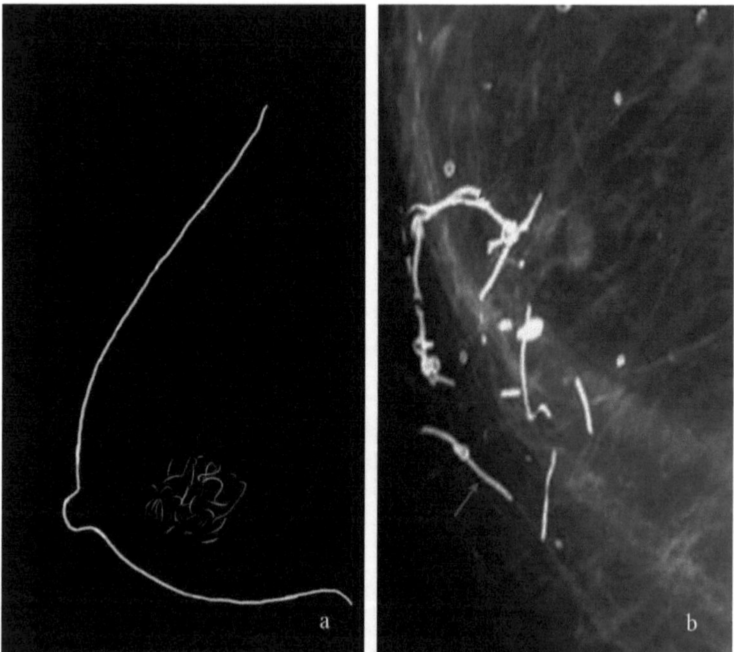

Fig. 35. Calcified sutures. (a) Diagram. (b) Mammogram. Linear calcifications along the suture path (arrows).

• **Dystrophic calcifications**

These calcifications usually appear in the irradiated breast, or after breast trauma. They are often irregular in shape, coarse and supra-millimetric (fig. 36).

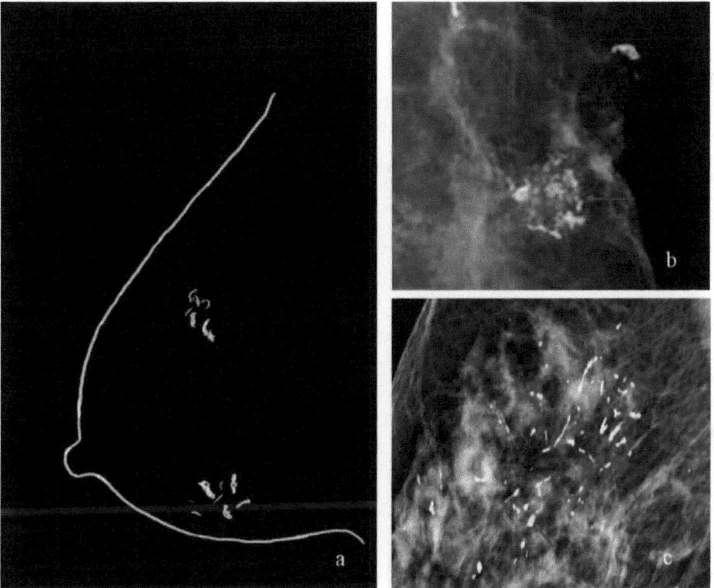

Fig. 36. Dystrophic calcifications. (a) Diagram. (b+c) Mammography. Irregular, coarse calcifications (arrows).

2.2.1.2. Calcifications suspected of malignancy

Four terms from the lexicon can be described: amorphous calcifications, coarse and heterogeneous calcifications, polymorphic fine calcifications and linear or branching fine calcifications.

- Amorphous microcalcifications

These are very fine calcifications, making it impossible to determine a specific form. When these calcifications are organized in isolated foci, they should be classified as BI-RADS 4b (10-50% malignancy), with a positive predictive value (PPV) of malignancy of 20% (fig. 27). The diffuse distribution of these microcalcifications may be benign.

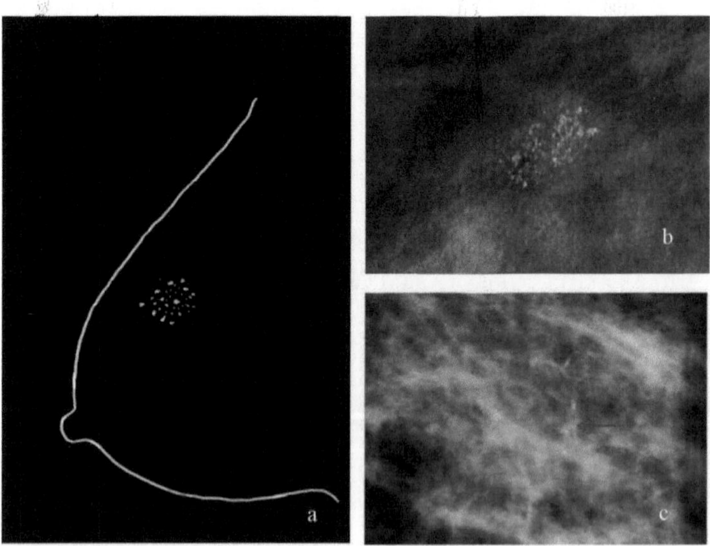

Fig. 37. Amorphous microcalcifications. (a) Diagram. (b+c) Mammography (b)

Focus of microcalcifications without specific shape (arrow). (c)

Linear microcalcifications with no specific shape (arrow).

- Coarse, heterogeneous microcalcifications

They correspond to irregular calcifications more often organized in clusters, between 0.5 and 1 mm in size, by definition smaller than dystrophic calcifications (> 1 mm) (fig. 38). They may be malignant or benign, and can be observed in fibroadenomas or cytosteonecrosis. In the case of isolated microcalcifications, they should be classified as BI-RADS 4b, with a PPV of malignancy of 15%.

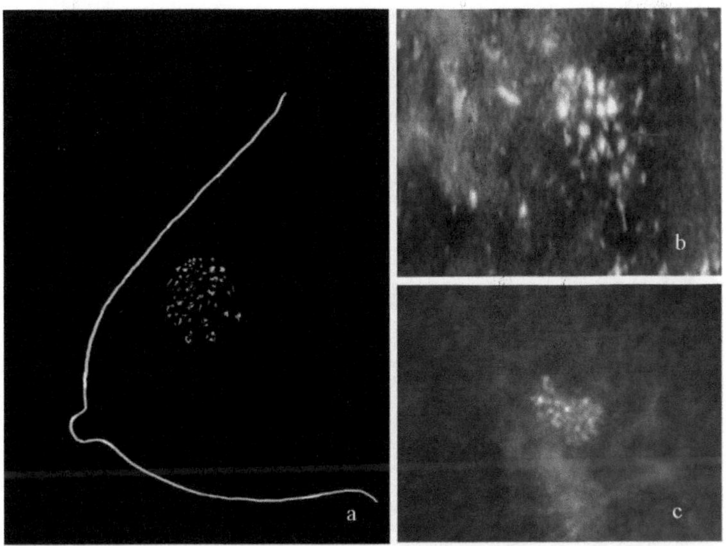

Fig. 38. Coarse, heterogeneous microcalcifications (a) Diagram. (b+c) Mammogram. (b) Focus of microcalcifications (arrow): non-specific infiltrating carcinoma (arrow). (c) Focus of microcalcifications: fibroadenoma (arrow).

- Fine polymorphic microcalcifications

They are generally more visible than amorphous calcifications, with no linear path (fig. 39). Their size and shape are irregular and variable, but usually less than 0.5 mm. They should be classified as BI-RADS 4b, with a PPV of 29%.

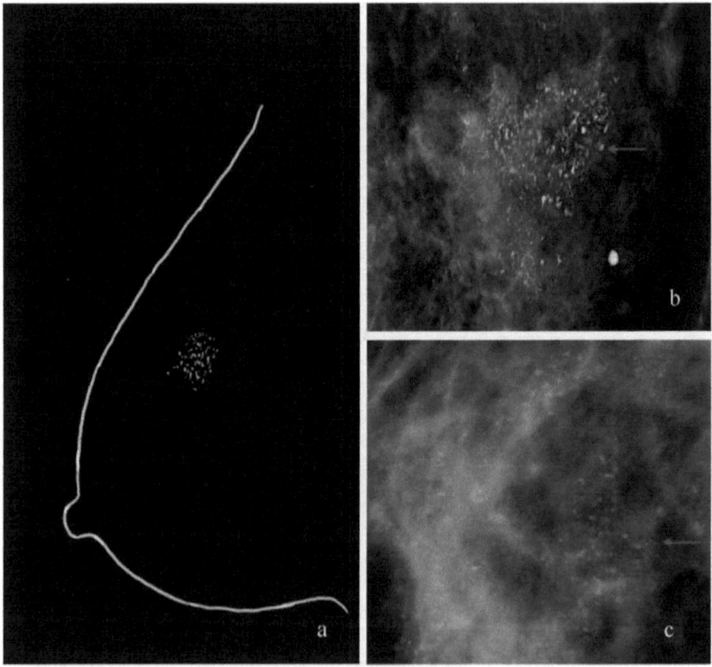

Fig. 39. Fine, polymorphic microcalcifications. (a) Schematic diagram. (b+c) Mammogram. Polymorphic, irregular microcalcifications (arrow): non-specific infiltrating carcinoma.

- Fine linear or branched calcifications

They are generally linear or irregularly curved, and less than 0.5 mm in size (fig. 40). Their morphology evokes the filling of a galactophore duct by tumor necrosis. They have a very high PPV of malignancy (70%) and, whatever their distribution, must be classified as at least BI-RADS 4c.

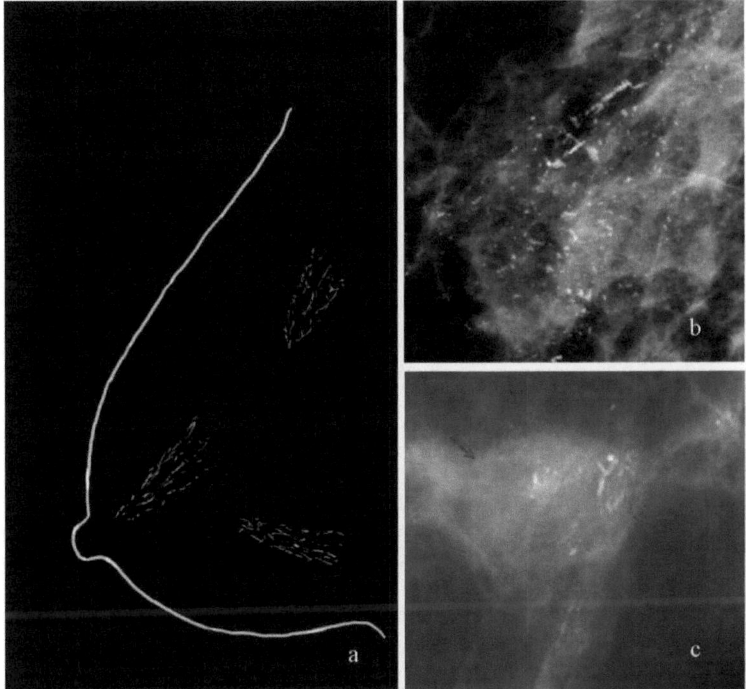

Fig. 40. Linear or branched fine calcifications. (a) Diagram. (b+c) Mammogram. Fine linear branching calcifications. (c) Irregular, spiculated mass associated with microcalcifications (arrows): non-specific infiltrating carcinoma.

2.2.2. Calcification distribution

The distribution of microcalcifications must also be analyzed. There are five types of distribution: diffuse, regional, clustered, linear and segmental.

2.2.2.1. Diffuse distribution

Calcifications are randomly and sparsely distributed in the breast, and are generally benign (fig. 41).

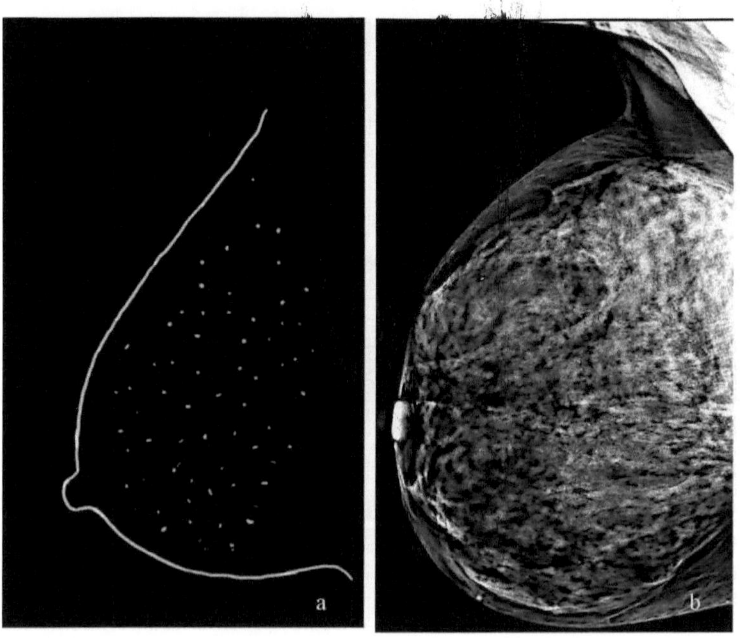

Fig. 41. Diffuse distribution (a) Diagram. (b) Mammogram. Scattered calcifications.

2.2.2.2. Regional distribution

These are calcifications grouped in a volume over 2 cm in diameter, but with no galactophoric orientation (fig. 42).

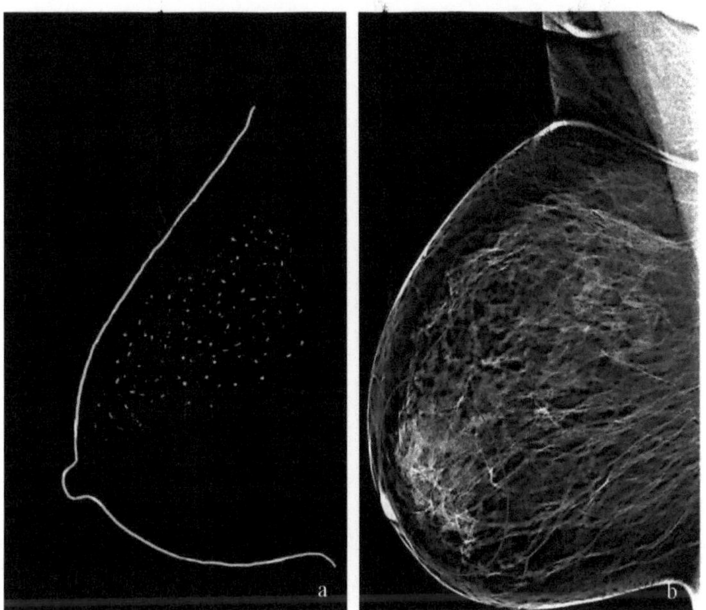

Fig. 42. Regional distribution. (a) Diagram. (b) Mammography. Calcifications in the retroareolar region (circle).

2.2.2.3. Group distribution

They correspond to a grouping of at least five microcalcifications within 1 cm and less than 2 cm (fig. 43).

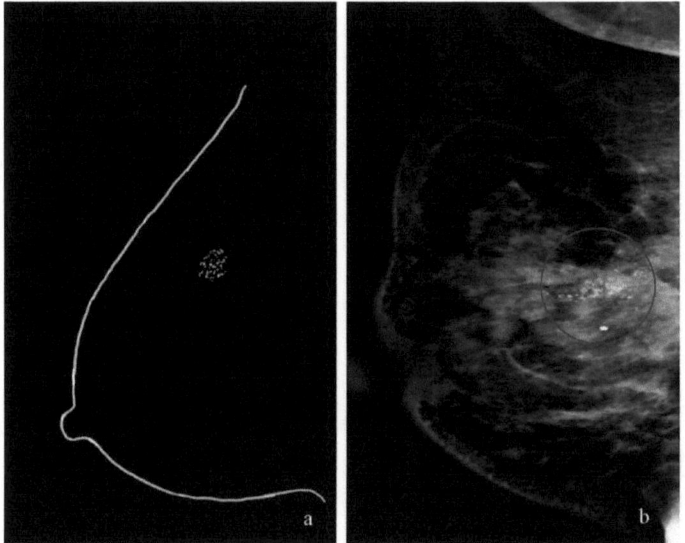

Fig. 43. Grouped distribution (a) Diagram. (b) Mammogram. Focus of microcalcifications extending over 2 cm (circle).

2.2.2.4. Linear distribution

These are calcifications with a galactophoric, linear course (fig. 44). This distribution is suggestive of intra-galactophoric calcium deposits, and its presence increases the suspicion of malignancy.

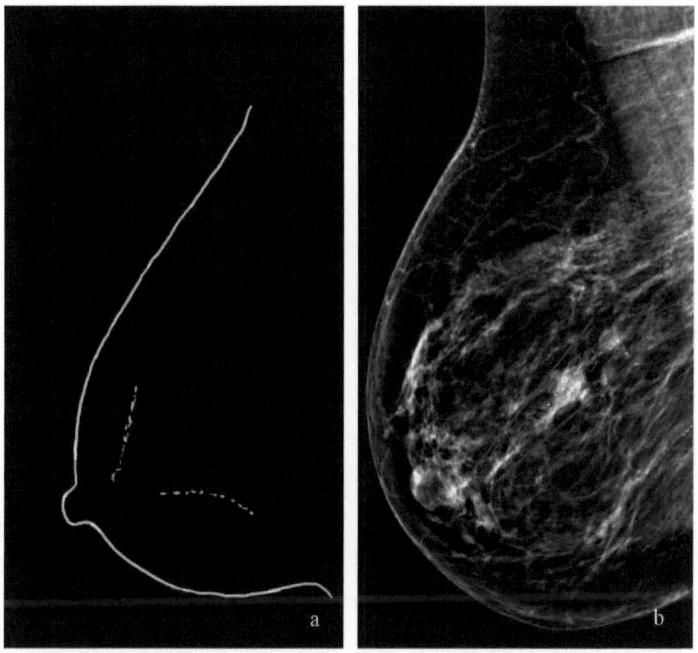

Fig. 44. Linear distribution. (a) Diagram. (b) Mammogram. Galactophoric tract calcifications.

2.2.2.5. Segmented distribution

Calcifications are triangular in distribution, with a peripheral base and apex converging towards the nipple (fig. 45).

Segmentally distributed calcifications are worrisome because they suggest calcium deposits in galactophore ducts, raising the possibility of extensive or multifocal breast carcinoma in a lobe or segment of the breast.

Benign segmental calcifications, such as secretory calcifications, can be differentiated from malignant, finer and more irregular calcifications of intra-canal carcinomas by their smooth rod morphology and large size.

A segmental distribution greatly increases the degree of suspicion for punctiform or amorphous calcifications, requiring histological examination.

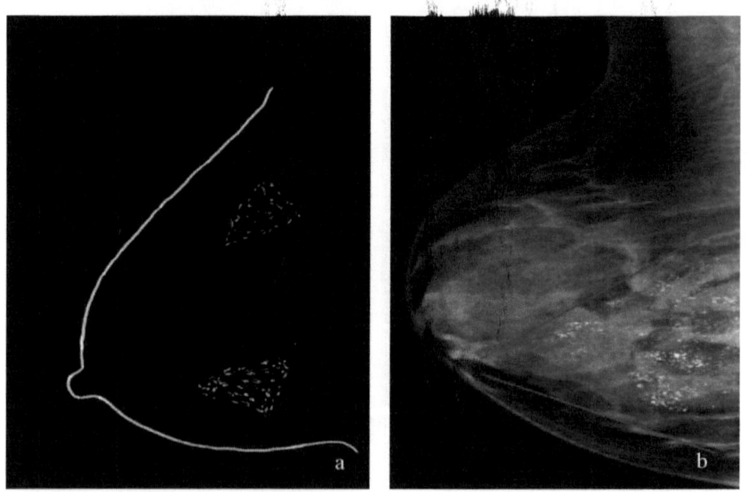

Fig. 45. Segment distribution. (a) Diagram. (b) Mammogram. Calcifications of triangular distribution, with peripheral base and apex converging towards the nipple.

The positive predictive values (PPV) of malignancy associated with
microcalcifications according to their morphology and distribution are
summarized in Table 3.

Table 3. Positive predictive values of malignancy associated with microcalcifications according to their morphology and distribution according to BI-RADS 2013.

Calcifications /Distribution Morphology	Diffuse (VPP = 0)	Regional, grouped (PPV: 26-31%)	Linear, segmented (PPV: 60-68%)
Round or punctiform	BI-RADS 2	BI-RADS 3	BI-RADS 4a
Heterogeneous coarse	BI-RADS 2	BI-RADS 4b	BI-RADS 4c
Amorphous or pleiomorphous	BI-RADS 2/3	BI-RADS 4b	BI-RADS 4c
Linear	BI-RADS 4a	BI-RADS 4c	BI-RADS 5

2.3. Architectural distortions

This is a break in the normal architecture of the breast parenchyma without a central mass, including fine lines or spicules radiating from a point. It may also be a focal reaction or distortion of the parenchymal margin. It may be associated with a mass, asymmetry or calcifications. In the absence of a history of trauma or surgery, this image is suspicious of malignancy or radial scarring, classified as BI-RADS 4c or 5 (fig. 46).

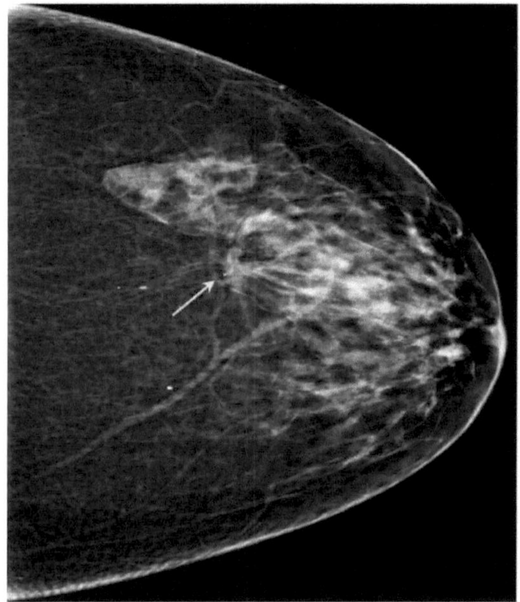

Fig. 46. Architectural distortion (arrow). Facing mammogram. Histology NST infiltrating carcinoma.

2.4. Density asymmetries

There are four types of density asymmetry. They may be visible on one or more incidences:

- **the asymmetry is visible on a single incidence** and corresponds to an area of fibro-glandular tissue, usually areas of glandular superimposition;
- **global asymmetry** is related to the presence of glandular tissue in comparison with the contralateral breast, occupying more than one quadrant;
- **focal asymmetry** is an anomaly that does not have the characteristics of a mass (density anomalies with concave edges and mixed with fat) and occupies less than one quadrant (fig. 47) ;
- **progressive asymmetry is** a density asymmetry of recent onset or modified compared with the previous examination. The PPV of malignancy for this anomaly is around 15%, and it should be classified as BI-RADS 4b.

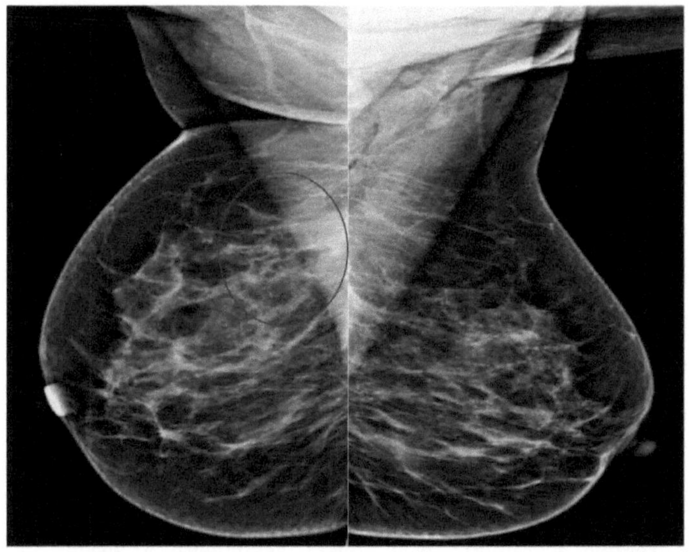

Fig. 47. Asymmetry of density (circle). Oblique mammogram. Histology, infiltrating carcinoma of NST.

2.5. Other

This chapter covers intramammary lymph nodes, skin lesions and isolated ductal dilatation. This last anomaly may sometimes be associated with a non-calcified intracanal cancer or papilloma, and should be classified as BI-RADS 4a, with a PPV of malignancy of 10%.

Other signs, isolated or associated with a mass, asymmetry or calcifications, include skin retraction, nipple retraction, skin thickening, trabecular thickening and axillary adenopathy (fig. 48).

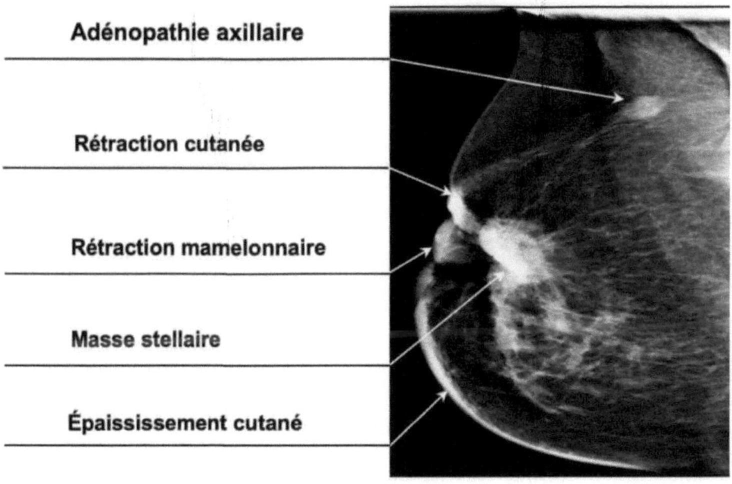

Fig. 48. Signs associated with a malignant mass.

3. Locating a lesion

A mammographic abnormality should be described according to the side of the breast, the quadrant and/or hourly radius, and the distance in centimetres from the nipple. A strict profile is required to specify the superior and inferior location of the lesion. Depth is described according to the three thirds of the breast: anterior, middle and posterior (fig. 49). A central lesion is located behind the nipple, a retroareolar lesion is located in the central part of the anterior third of the breast, and an axillary extension lesion in the upper part of the superolateral quadrant.

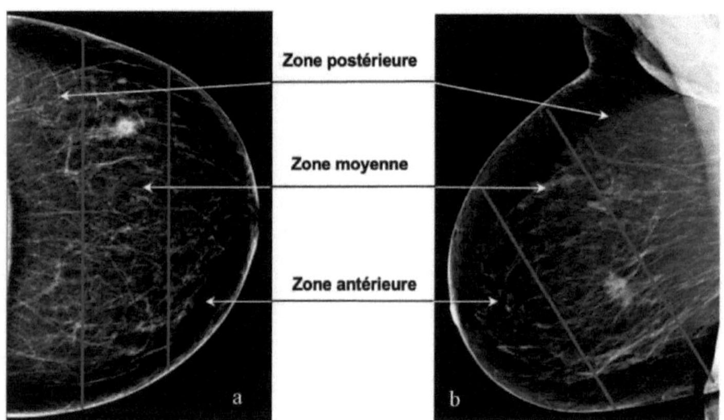

Fig. 49. Deep topography of the mass. (a) Mammography, front view (b) Mammography, oblique view. Example, mass located in the middle mammary region.

4. Malignancy probability score

The BI-RADS 0 category is reserved only for incomplete examinations, if additional images such as enlargements, localized centric views or ultrasound exploration are missing. BI-RADS 0 classification may be chosen provisionally in the absence of previous mammographic images for comparison. Finally, a BI-RADS 0 mammogram should not be classified while waiting for a breast MRI. However, the appropriate category should be used, e.g. BIRADS 4 if an abnormality is suspected.

BI-RADS 1 or 2 categories, no anomalies or benign anomalies.

The BI-RADS 3 category reflects a probably benign abnormality requiring short-term surveillance, with a probability of malignancy of between 0 and 2%. This category includes three types of mammographic anomalies:
- a solid mass with regular contours and no calcification;
- focal density asymmetry with concave boundaries and/or mixed with fat;
- an isolated cluster of punctiform microcalcifications.

Surveillance of a BI-RADS 3 abnormality on mammography is as follows: unilateral check at 6 months, bilateral check at 1 year, then check at 2 or even 3 years. If the abnormality is stable at 2 or 3 years, it is reclassified as BI-RADS 2.

BI-RADS 4 means an undetermined abnormality requiring biopsy. BI-RADS 4 has a broad cancer PPV of between 2% and 95%, and we recommend using the sub-categories BI-RADS 4a, BI-RADS 4b and BI-RADS 4c. A BI-RADS 4a lesion with a cancer PPV of between 2% and 10%. It includes amorphous or dusty calcifications, grouped in clusters.

A lesion classified as BI-RADS 4b with a PPV of cancer between 10 and 50%. These may be dusty or amorphous microcalcifications with segmental distribution, coarse heterogeneous microcalcifications in clusters, or a solid mass with indistinct contours.

A BI-RADS 4c lesion has a PPV of cancer of 50-95%. The following abnormalities can be classified as BI-RADS 4c: a newly appeared solid mass with indistinct contours, architectural distortion outside a known and stable scar, a new focus of fine linear microcalcifications.

The BI-RADS 5 category is suggestive of cancer, with a PPV > 95%; it includes the following abnormalities: a mass with a blurred or irregular contour, a mass with a spiculated contour, fine linear or fine branched linear microcalcifications. The lesion requires histological verification.

BI-RADS 6 means histologically proven cancer.

ACR BI-RADS mammography classification

The ACR BI-RADS classification is summarized in Table 4 [1].

Classification of mammographic abnormalities	
Level BI-RADS	ACR BI-RADS classification Mammography and treatment guidelines (CAT)
BI-RADS 0	**Mammography pending further diagnosis**
BI-RADS 1	**Normal mammography**
BI-RADS 2	**Anomalies considered benign (PPV of cancer = 0%)** • Round masses with coarse calcifications (adenofibroma or cyst). • Intramammary ganglion. • Round mass corresponding to a typical cyst on ultrasound. • Mixed density mass (lipoma, hamartoma, galactocele, oily cyst). • Known scar. • Cutaneous and vascular calcifications. • Large, light-centered, parietal, milk-calcium-type, dystrophic, rod-shaped calcifications, calcified sutures. • Diffuse regular round calcifications.

BI-RADS 3	**Anomalies considered probably benign (PPV of cancer < 2%)** **CAT: short-term monitoring 4 to 6 months recommended** • Sparse, round or amorphous calcifications in small, isolated clusters. • Small round or oval cluster of polymorphous calcifications, few in number, suggestive of incipient adenofibroma calcification. • Well-circumscribed, round, oval or discreetly polycyclic mass without microlobulation, non-calcified, non-fluid on ultrasound. • Focal asymmetry of density with concave boundaries and/or mixed with fat.
BI-RADS 4	**Anomalies considered suspicious (PPV > 2% and < 95%)** **CAT: biopsy.** • Numerous round calcifications and/or clusters with neither round nor oval outlines. • Amorphous or dusty calcifications, grouped and numerous. • Heterogeneous coarse calcifications or few fine polymorphic calcifications. • Architectural distortion outside a known, stable scar. • Round or oval non-fluid mass with microlobulated contours, or masked by normal fibroglandular tissue, or which has increased in volume. • Focal density asymmetry with convex or progressive boundaries.

BI-RADS 4a	**Low probability of malignancy; CAT: biopsy.** - Amorphous or dusty calcifications, grouped in clusters.
BI-RADS 4b	**Intermediate probability of malignancy; CAT: biopsy.** • Amorphous or dusty calcifications, segmentally distributed. • Heterogeneous coarse calcifications in clusters.

BI-RADS 4c	**Moderate probability of malignancy; CAT: biopsy.** - Architectural distortion outside a known, stable scar.
BI-RADS 5	**Anomalies considered malignant (PPV > 95%)** **CAT: biopsy and multidisciplinary management.** • Fine linear or fine branched calcifications. • Coarse, heterogeneous calcifications or fine, polymorphous calcifications, numerous and grouped in clusters. • Grouped calcifications of any morphology, with linear or segmental distribution (intragalactophoric topography). • Calcifications associated with architectural distortion or mass. • Clustered calcifications that have increased in number or calcifications whose morphology and distribution have become more suspect. • A mass with a blurred or irregular contour. • Spiculated contour mass.

BI-RADS 6	**Known cancer, biopsy-proven malignancy** **CAT: biopsy and multidisciplinary management.**

References

1. D'Orsi CJ et al. ACR BI-RADS Atlas, Breast Imaging Reporting and Data System. Reston, VA, American College of Radiology; 2013.

2. Couturaud B, Fitoussi A. Anatomy/surgery of breast cancer. Conservative treatment, oncoplasty. Techniques chirurgicales gynécologie. Elsevier Masson; 2011; 4-7.

3. Baur A, Bahrs SD, Speck S, Wietek BM, Kremer B, Vogel U, et al. Breast MRI of pure ductal carcinoma in situ: sensitivity of diagnosis and influence of lesion characteristics. Eur J Radiol 2013;82:1731-7.

4. Hammersleya JA, Partridgeb SC, Blitzera GC, Deitcha S, Rahbarb H. Management of high-risk breast lesions found on mammogram or ultrasound: the value of contrast-enhanced MRI to exclude malignancy. Clinical Imaging 49; 2018; 174180.

5. Andolina VF, Lillé SL, Willison KM, Mammographic Imaging. A pratical guide. 2 nd ed. Lippincott Williams and Wilkins; 2001.

6. Austin C. R and Short R. V. Hormonal Control of Reproduction. 2nd edition of Reproduction in Mammals, Vol.3. Cambridge : Cambridge University Press. 1984.

7. Faulconer LS, Parham CA, Connor DM, Kuzmiak C, et al. Effect of breast compression on lesion characteristic visibility with diffraction-enhanced imaging. Acad Radiol 2010; 17 (4) : 433-40. Epub 2009 Dec 29.

8. Kinzelin S. Positioning, the key step in mammography examination. Imagerie du sein Elsevier Masson, 2012; 2: 19-27.

9. Mancuso S, Ottolenghi G. The oblique projection in the radiologic Study of the breast. Minerva Ginecol 1989; 41 (7): 325-8.

10. Konguth PJ, Rimer BK, Conaway MR, et al. Impact of patient-controlled compression on the mammography experience. Radiology 1993; 186 (1) : 99-102.

11. Muntz EP, Logan WW, Focal spot size. And scatter supression in magnification mammography. AJR Am J Roentgenol 1979; 133 (3) : 453-9.

12. Heywang-Kobrunner S H, Schreer I, Bassler R, Perlet C, Viehweg P. Normal breast. Imagerie diagnostique du sein : Mammographie, échographie, IRM, techniques interventionnelles 2007 ; 183-202.

13. Chopier J, Salem C, Billières P, Balleyguier C. Variation of the normal breast: mammographic and ultrasonographic aspects. Encycl Méd Chir 2003; 34-800-A-15.

14. Goumot PA, Bremond A, Dilhuydy MH, et al. La lecture mammographique : Sémiologie le sein normal. Le Sein : Son Image 1993.

15. Tabar L, Dean PB. Basic principals of mammogtaphic diagnosis. Diagn Imaging Clin Med 1985; 54 (3-4).

16. Meyer JE, Ferraro FA, Frenna TH, Di Piro PJ, Denison CM. Mammographic appearance of normal intramammary lymph nodes in an atypical location. AJR Am J Roentgenol 1993; 161: 779-780.

17. Wolfe JN. Astudy of breast parenchyma by mammography in the normal woman and those with benign and malignant disease of the breast. Radiology 1967; 89: 210-215

18. Davros WJ, Madsen EL, Zagzebski JA. Breast mass detection by US: a phantom study. Radiology 1985; 156: 773-775.

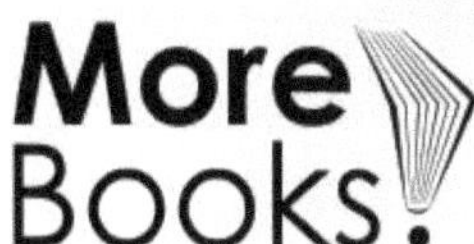
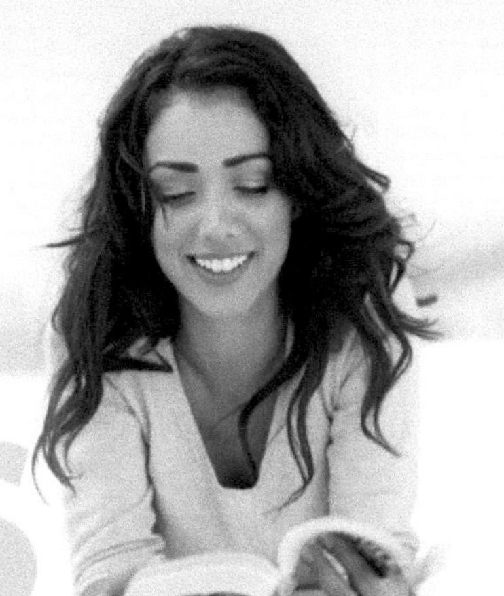